Tania Felipe Reyes

Elements Of Community Nursing

Tania Felipe Reyes

Elements Of Community Nursing

Quality in primary nursing care

ScienciaScripts

Imprint

Any brand names and product names mentioned in this book are subject to trademark, brand or patent protection and are trademarks or registered trademarks of their respective holders. The use of brand names, product names, common names, trade names, product descriptions etc. even without a particular marking in this work is in no way to be construed to mean that such names may be regarded as unrestricted in respect of trademark and brand protection legislation and could thus be used by anyone.

Cover image: www.ingimage.com

This book is a translation from the original published under ISBN 978-620-3-03492-9.

Publisher:
Sciencia Scripts
is a trademark of
International Book Market Service Ltd., member of OmniScriptum Publishing Group
17 Meldrum Street, Beau Bassin 71504, Mauritius
Printed at: see last page
ISBN: 978-620-3-33242-1

ELEMENTS OF COMMUNITY NURSING

Author: Tania Felipe

Reyes Bachelor's

Degree in Nursing

1st Degree Specialist in Community Nursing

Assistant Professor of the Faculty of Medical Sciences of Sancti Spiritus Cuba.

Collaborators

Msc. Msc Maria Elena Pacheco Sosa

Eng. Ms.C Benigno Leyva de la Cruz

Eng.

DEDICATION

This book is dedicated to nursing professionals working in primary health care, nursing students and teachers.

PREFACE

The diversity of community health topics was the reason for the elaboration of this text whose purpose is to unify important contents for the community professional as a guide for daily work. The book is intended for all nursing students, teachers and professionals working in primary health care. It describes in a dynamic and entertaining way the different work algorithms in community work.

For its preparation, national and international bibliographic reviews have been carried out, extracting the useful aspects for community work. Taking into account methodological aspects of the contents for the accessible assimilation of these contents.

The use of this text favors the organized work of the community charge nurse and the preparation of a competent professional for the performance of community work.

INDEX

Collaborators 1

DEDICATION 2

PREFACE 2

CHAPTER 1: 5

EMERGENCE OF COMMUNITY NURSING 5

1.1   Mission and vision 6

1.2   Roles of the community nurse 6

1.3   Characteristics of community care 7

CHAPTER 2: 8

TRANSCULTURAL NURSING 8

2.1   Concept of transcultural nursing 8

2.2   Ethical principles of the nursing professional in transculturation 9

2.3   Nursing theory underpinning transculturation of community care nurses 11

CHAPTER 3: 13

THE HOME VISIT 13

3.1   Objectives 13

3.2   Structure or stages 13

3.3   Requirements for an effective visit 15

3.4   Case technique 16

CHAPTER 4: 20

PALLIATIVE CARE FOR PATIENTS IN THE COMMUNITY 20

4.1   Nursing theory underpinning the palliative work of the nursing professional in the community 21

4.2   Objectives of palliative care 21

4.3   Needs of a palliative care patient 21

4.4   Bed bath procedure 22

4.5   Morning and evening care procedure 25

4.6   Feeding procedure for a palliative care patient 26

CHAPTER 5: 33

COMMUNICATION 33

5.1 Factors that distort communication 34

5.2 Health communication techniques 36

CHAPTER 6: 38

COMMUNITY HEALTH PROMOTION AND PREVENTION 38

6.1 Nursing fields of action in health education 39

CHAPTER 7: 41

SYNTHESIS OF NURSING THEORIES AND MODELS APPLIED TO
COMMUNITY CARE 41

7.1 Types of models 41

7.2 Florence Nightingale's theory 42

7.3 Virginia Henderson's model 42

7.4 M o d e l o f Dorothea Orem 43

7.5 Peplau Model 45

7.6 Callista Roy Model 45

7.7 Martha Rogers' model 47

CHAPTER 8: 48

ACCIDENTS IN THE HOME 48

8.1 Most common accidents 48

8.2 General causes 49

8.3 Activities to prevent accidents in the home 50

8.4 The community health professional's role in accident prevention 52

BIBLIOGRAPHY 55

CHAPTER 1:
EMERGENCE OF COMMUNITY NURSING

Community nursing was born with the creation of the Ministry of Health and social assistance and valuing the family as a working unit, this situation determined that each nurse was assigned a certain number of families and communities in their care. Community nursing is the part of nursing that develops and applies in an integral way, within the framework of public health, the care of the individual, the family and the community in health and illness. Community nursing is a synthesis of nursing practice and public health applied to promote and preserve the health of the population. The nature of this practice is general and encompasses many aspects. It is continuous and contributes to improving the health of the population as a whole. Nursing care in the community goes back to the knowledge of life itself and the notion of human survival, it focuses on the health needs of the population, throughout the life of the individual. Community nursing is the part of nursing that develops and applies comprehensive care to families and communities in the unstable balance between health and disease. It specifically contributes to individuals, families and communities acquiring skills, habits and behaviors that promote self-care within the framework of primary health care, which includes health promotion, protection, recovery, prevention and rehabilitation.

Health problems and needs must be approached from a quality and interdisciplinary perspective. Community nursing should be an advocate for values that contribute to maintaining greater solidarity and social justice, and equality of opportunity. The community nurse should monitor health in the community as a whole and determine the impact of their actions on groups or sets of groups served in relation to the total community and their level of health. The community nurse reorients and empowers individuals, families and communities to care for themselves and is able to transform dependency into self-care.

It has its antecedents in the English Sanitary Movement of the 19th century, following the Chadwick report (1837).

William Rathbone and Florence Nightingale.

In the 20th century, the health visitor system was developed.

It also spread to other countries in Europe and the United States, leading to the creation of schools.

1.1 Mission and vision

The vision of the community nurse to society is expressed as an integral service in all care processes with the vision of the nursing process as a work tool and with care practice based on scientific evidence.

The mission is to help individuals, families and communities to determine and achieve their physical, mental and social potential and to realize it within the environment in which they live and work.

1.2 Roles of the community nurse

The personnel that assists the community environment and endowed with all the ethical and moral principles that the profession requires develops professional skills that facilitate the best development of the assigned task and have the responsibility to go through all the activities entrusted to the nursing professional.

- Assistance: Refers to the work carried out in the health institution and in the community, pursuing the preventive, curative and rehabilitation of individuals, families and the community.
- Teacher: The health professional carries out health promotion activities using methodological aspects that make it possible to achieve the understanding of the different topics, in addition to collaborating in the training of the new generation.
- Administration: The nursing professional performs administrative control of equipment, accessories medications that are under his/her custody for patient care, as well as coordinates activities of the health team.
- Researcher: In order to improve the quality of patient care, the nursing

professional must be updated on health and care issues, which is why it is necessary to be involved in research.

In the scientific community, the annual health situation analysis is one of the most important

The main epidemiological research carried out by community care personnel is an inseparable tool for community work.

1.3 Characteristics of community care

In order to achieve the proposed purpose or objective, community care must meet a number of qualities that make the work is done optimally, involving different sectors that from their radius of action provide benefits for the implementation of actions aimed at the same purpose such as:

- Integrator
- Continuous and permanent
- Activate
- Accessible
- Multidisciplinary
- Participatory
- Programmed
- Evaluable
- Teacher
- Researcher

CHAPTER 2:
TRANSCULTURAL NURSING

The relationship between culture and nursing and anthropology is long and extensive. Each individual internalizes and applies care according to his or her culture, that is to say, according to his or her customs, values, beliefs, and since the beginning of the world, these techniques have somehow served as a means of survival. This situation is confirmed by the development of transcultural nursing where cultural competence is considered a necessary condition for nursing care in all patients.

Nurses must be careful to be discerning with respect to personal cultural values and beliefs and separate them from the values and beliefs of the patients with whom they are dealing. In order to provide culturally sensitive care, the nurse must remember that each individual is unique and is the product of beliefs, customs, and values passed down from one generation to the next. Awareness and acceptance of cultural differences is an exercise that involves the actions of the nurse. We should not fall into paternalistic behaviors or, on the contrary, but rather care for the person from another culture as we would care for any other person, respecting individual differences and focusing on the quality of the humanized service we are providing. The area of transcultural nursing involves avoiding stereotypes and overcoming prejudices in order to establish an effective relationship with the user, accepting cultural differences.

2.1 Concept of transcultural nursing

It is based on an ideology as a way of focusing care towards cultural consideration in its practice, as stated by Lenninger is nothing more than providing care that is consistent with the culture to give quality to it and for this, the individual culture must be known in order to be applied. Transculturally trained nurses must take into account cultural beliefs, caring behaviors and values of individuals individually, as well as families and the different social groups in their care to provide effective, satisfactory and consistent care with the objective of developing a body of humanized and scientific knowledge to provide a culturally specific and universal nursing practice. Transcultural nursing: refers to nurses who are trained in transcultural nursing and whose task is to develop transcultural nursing knowledge and practice.

Cross-cultural nursing : Refers to nurses who use medical or applied anthropological concepts; most are not authorized to develop transcultural nursing theory or conduct research-based practice.

2.2 Ethical principles of the nursing professional in transculturation.

Compliance with the ethical principles of nursing is of vital importance to achieve the objectives proposed by the community nurse.

1. Beneficence: benevolence or non-maleficence, ethical principle of doing good and avoiding harm or evil to oneself or to society. Acting with benevolence means helping others to obtain what is beneficial to them, or that promotes their well-being, reducing maleficent risks, which may cause them physical or psychological harm.

2. Autonomy: ethical principle that advocates the individual freedom that each person has to determine his or her own actions, according to his or her choice. Respecting people as autonomous individuals means recognizing their decisions, made in accordance with their personal values and convictions. One of the problems in the application of the principle of autonomy in nursing care is that the patient may have different levels of capacity to make an autonomous decision, depending on his or her internal limitations (mental aptitude, level of consciousness, age or health condition) or external limitations (hospital environment, availability of existing resources, amount of information provided for making an informed decision, among others).

3. Justice: once the ways of practicing beneficence have been determined, the nurse needs to be concerned with how to distribute these benefits or resources among his or her patients, such as the disposition of his or her time and care among the various patients according to the needs that arise. Justice is the principle of being equitable or fair, that is, equal treatment among equals and differential treatment among unequals, according to individual need. This means that people with equal health needs should receive equal quantity and quality of services and resources. And people with greater needs than others should receive more services than others according to need. The principle of justice is closely related to the principles of fidelity and truthfulness.

4. Fidelity: principle of building trust between the professional and the patient. It is, in fact, an obligation or commitment to be faithful in the relationship with the patient, in which the nurse must keep promises and maintain reliability. The patient's expectation is that professionals will keep their word. Only in exceptional circumstances, when the benefits of breaking the promise outweigh keeping it, can the promise be broken. Trust is the basis for spontaneous confidence, and facts revealed in confidence are part of the nurse's professional secret.

5. Truthfulness: ethical principle of always telling the truth, not lying and not deceiving patients. In many cultures, truthfulness has been considered the basis for establishing and maintaining trust between individuals. An of cultural variation would be on the quality of information to be provided in relation to diagnosis and treatment. Thus, it may be difficult to develop a form to obtain consent from a patient who has not been informed of his or her diagnosis.

The practitioner should assess the importance for the participant to know his or her diagnosis in relation to the intended treatment or care.

6. Confidentiality: ethical principle of safeguarding personal information obtained during the exercise of his or her function as a nurse and maintaining the professional secrecy of this information, not communicating to anyone the personal confidences made by patients.

Ethics and values are unavoidable principles that should characterize nursing professionals, which demands respect, dignity to life, quality, efficiency, beneficence, truthfulness, and justice towards the patient to whom care is given.

2.3 Nursing theory underpinning the transculturation of the community care nursing workforce.

Madeleine Leininger

"Cultural care: theory of diversity and universality."

Leininger, the founder of transcultural nursing and a leader in the theory of caring for people in transcultural nursing, was the first college-prepared nurse practitioner to win an award in cultural and social anthropology. She was born in Sutton Nebraska and began her nursing career after graduating from St. Anthony's Denver School of   Nursing.

Theoretical sources

Leininger drew on the discipline of anthropology and nursing defined transcultural nursing as a major area of nursing that focuses on the comparative study and analysis of different cultures and subcultures of the world with respect to values about care, expression and beliefs of health and illness, and behavioral modeling, whose purpose is to devise a scientific and humanistic knowledge to provide culture-specific nursing care practice and
a universal nursing care practice of the culture.
Transcultural nursing goes beyond knowledge and makes use of cultural

nursing care knowledge to practice culturally congruent and responsible care Leininger states that over time there will be a new type of nursing practice that will reflect the different types of nursing, which will be defined and based on culture and will be specific to guide nursing care directed at individuals, families, groups, and institutions. Afirma that culture and care are the broadest means of conceptualizing and understanding people this knowledge is essential for nursing education and practice.

Leininger defines that, as well as nursing is significative for patients and for nurses around the world the knowledge of transcultural nursing and its competencies will be essential to guide the decisions and actions of nurses and thus obtain good and eficient results able to apply general concepts principles and practices of transcultural nursing created by transcultural nurse specialists on the other hand Leinninger defines and promotes a new and different theory, and not traditional nursing theory, which is usually defined as a set of logically related concepts and hypothetical propositions that can be tested in order to explain or predict a fact, phenomenon or situation. In contrast, Leininger defines theory as the systematic and creative discovery of knowledge of a field of interest or phenomenon that seems relevant to understanding or explaining unknown phenomena.

Leininger, created the theory of diversity and universality of cultural nursing care, which has its foundations in the belief that people from different cultures can inform and guide professionals and thus, they will be able to receive the type of health care they want and need from these professionals. Cultures represent the systematized patterns of their lives and the values of the people who influence their

Therefore, the theory is focused on nurses discovering and acquiring knowledge about the patient's world and making use of their internal views, their knowledge.

CHAPTER 3:
THE HOME VISIT

The home visit is the set of social and health activities provided at home to people. This care allows to detect, assess, support and control the health problems of the individual and the family, enhancing autonomy and improving the quality of life of people, is considered the basic activity of the nurse in the sense of solving health problems and crises of the individual, family and community, allowing actions to promote and prevent health to achieve healthy lifestyles, allows healing, rehabilitation and incorporation into society.The home visit is a strategy for the delivery of health services at home directed to families framed in a plan of action defined by the health team, allowing health interventions in the context of people's lives.

3.1 Objectives

1- The purpose of the home visit is to verify the composition of the family nucleus, socioeconomic level of the individual, distribution of social spaces, personal and family behavior, family health and relevant aspects to be evaluated as they have a direct impact on the population in their care, contributing to improve the quality of life through integrated and coordinated actions for health promotion, prevention and rehabilitation.

2- To strengthen environmental actions and family ties that favor the biopsychosocial development of the population.

3- Extend care coverage to all members of the family group.

4- Improve the use of available resources through the application of protocols according to age groups, pathologies and needs.

3.2 Structure or stages

Planning: This is done by the health team, date, time and objective are coordinated.

Introduction: Explain to the family the purpose of the visit, being important the rapport that must be created by the nurse in order to achieve a climate of trust and security between nurse, family, patient.

Development: It is divided for its better development in 3 stages. Work is done on the aspects that motivated the visit.

1- Home tour: Risk factors are identified, family functioning test (FF-SIL test) is performed.

2- General physical examination of the individual

3- Observation of environmental hygiene risks in the community.

Conclusions: It is the summary of the most important aspects by elaborating an action plan to be followed by the family in the absence of the nurse, recommendations are left and the next visit is coordinated.

The estimated time of the home visit will depend on the family situation and the objectives set. It should be approximately 20 to 30 minutes.

Evaluation of the home visit: An analysis is carried out by the members of the health team to evaluate the fulfillment of the proposed objectives.

Types of home visits

- First contact: it is carried out for the first time in the home, arises from an initial intervention is carried out to establish the first contact.

- Follow-up visits: These are part of an intervention plan and evaluation objectives set.

- Epidemiological visit: Aimed at conducting an epidemiological investigation of apathology under surveillance.

- Patient rescue or summons: We go to the patient's home to summon them for a specific health task or to find out if they are absent for an appointment.

- Unsuccessful visit: When you go to the home and you are unable to have contact with the family.

Advantages of the home visit
✓ It allows to observe the family in its environmental and social environment.

✓ The family actively participates

✓ Allows the nurse to be aware of the social and environmental characteristics of the families in her care.

Qualities of human resources

✓ Training and education

✓ Professional Experience

✓ Ability to relate

✓ Provide relevant information at the right time

✓ Ability to develop trusting relationships with family members, interest and commitment to the task.

3.3 Requirements for an effective visit

The family environment requires privacy on the part of its members; therefore, the nursing professional has the obligation to establish behavioral guidelines, ethical elements and professional development that will allow him/her to efficiently perform this community practice.

• Need of the family or individual: Working with the felt needs of thepopulation allows the professional to have accessibility to the family and to the achievement of the objectives.

• Pathological history: If the nursing staff is visiting the patient for the first time, they should make a broad anamnesis with emphasis on family and personal pathological history that will allow them to work with the risk factors and thus prevent the disease from being triggered.

• Housing conditions: The conditions for an effective visit should be created in advance, e.g. pets should be protected to avoid injury to health personnel, rooms should be well lit and ventilated, and a room should be available to allow the physical examination and the conclusions of the visit to be made.

• Sanitary facilities and cultural environment. The health personnel will create a favorable environment to facilitate family exchanges and to ensure that the interview and other community procedures are carried out in a fruitful manner.

3.4 Briefcase technique

Through the use of the briefcase, the nurse provides teaching in an indirect way, the family observes with attention the information provided, specific equipment and materials are used, serving as motivation.

Briefcase technique

Objectives: To carry basic equipment to provide nursing care in the home or other setting as needed.

Provide nursing care, including techniques and demonstrations. Procedure:

Before going out to the field, prepare the briefcase according to the planning of your home visit and probable situations that may arise, depending on the family, school, kindergarten, company, etc. to be visited. In order to carry out an effective home visit, you must take into account that you will need an adequate briefcase with all the necessary items.

Through the use of the briefcase the nurse provides teaching in an indirect way; the family observes carefully the information provided, specific equipment and materials are used.

Contents of the case:

Its content is variable, depending on the type of interverventionstobe carried out, except for the transfer of biological products, which should be placed in thermoses recommended in the universal vaccination program.

Instruments

• Strong clamp (Rochester)

Team

- Sterile and non-sterile test tube in suficient quantity.

- Rectal or axillary clinical thermometer

- Baumanometer

- Pinard stethoscope

- Portfolio with home visit request forms and educational material.

Consumables

Basic Equipment:1 briefcase

1 bottle with alcohol (60 to 100cc)

1 bottle with alcohol hand wash gel dry if necessary 3 ampoules of

serum fisiological 20cc.

1 bottle with liquid soap

1 scissors

3 low tongues or disposable depressors

1 bottle with dry cotton swabs (large and small) nova towel 1 plastic breastplate 1 nylon 0.50 cm x 0.50 cm

1 piece of paper 0.50 cm x 0.50 cm (kraft or white paper type, not printed) Paper or plastic bags for waste.

1 measuring rod

Non-sterile disposable gloves

1 esfigmomanometer with

stethoscope 1 flashlight

1 thermometer

1 small clean kidney (to place the thermometer)

1 monofilamento (piece of fishing line)

1 small file cabinet with set of educational materials

Depending on the need, material will be added to the basic equipment to perform specific techniques, such as cures, taking urine and blood tests at home, material for DSM stimulation, weight, etc.

Basic technique for the use of the

 briefcase Steps:

1. Choose a flat, sturdy, safe and comfortable place; hold the wallet and the case with one hand: take out the plastic frame from between the flaps and the lid and spread it on the chosen place.

2. Place the briefcase on a paper field on the left side.

3. Wash hands with running water or ask the family for a container of clean water.

4. Dry your m a n s w i t   h t h e p ap e ly towel and dispose of it in the waste bag.

5. Open the case.

6. Take out of the briefcase the material and equipment to be used and place it in a clean field.

7. Performs the necessary activities and procedures by carrying them out in an orderly manner.

8. Make the necessary annotations.

9. Store the material and equipment in the case in an orderly manner.

10. Discard   in the bag of material used during used during the procedures as well as the paper field.

11. Closes the case perfectly.

Case for nursing home visits, especially designed to transport medical material, being of the type consisting of a prismatic body (2), provided with support blocks (3) at its lower base (4), as well as a handle (5), characterized by the fact that the aforementioned.

CHAPTER 4:

PALLIATIVE CARE FOR PATIENTS IN THE COMMUNITY

Palliative home care allows people to remain in their own homes to receive end-of-life care. at these times, families require outside help. Hence, many of them opt for caregivers with expertise in palliative nursing and care. In end-of-life palliative care, nurses take on roles ranging from pain management and symptom control to assessing coping mechanisms for both the patient and family and providing them with the resources available to assist them.

According to the WHO, palliative care is appropriate for the patient with advanced and progressive disease where the control of pain and other symptoms, as well as psychosocial and spiritual aspects become more important.

In the integral care of the patient in the advanced stage of the disease in his residence. It has great advantages and some disadvantages for the patient and for the family. It is the essence of palliative care and with well-formed teams it is possible to give good quality of life and dignified death to patients with advanced terminal illness.

Advantages for the patient

They maintain their social and family role, have their own time and distribute it, maintain their privacy and occupational activities for the patient and family, are in a familiar environment, have the affection of their family and it has been proven that there is an increase in the quality of life with respect to hospitalized patients.

Advantages for the family

Familiar environment, ease of movement, time, satisfaction with active participation in care, facilitation of the grieving process, respect for the patient's wishes.

4.1 Nursing theory underpinning the palliative work of the nursing professional in the community.

Dorothea Orem's general theory is made up of 3 interrelated theories: Self-care theory

Self-care deficit theory Nursing

systems theory Other theories

such as:

 Jean Watson's theory

Florence Nightingale's

theory Calista Roy's theory.

4.2 Objectives of palliative care

The goal of palliative care is to achieve the best quality of life for the patient and his or her family, to obtain a dignified death. Palliative curative treatments are not mutually exclusive, but a matter of emphasis.

4.3 Needs of a palliative care patient

Taking into account the basic needs for the preservation of life and the hierarchical elements of Kalish's pyramid, the community nurse will identify in each patient which are the needs that appear in each stage of palliative care, as well as the technical elements that each need must meet to achieve the goals set, we refer to the following needs:

❖ Hygiene, rest and sleep needs

❖ Nutritional needs

❖ Urinary elimination needs

❖ Intestinal elimination needs.

❖ Oxygen requirements

❖ Need for security and self-esteem.

4.4 Bed bath procedure

Shower bath). It is the bath that is done under running water, with the help of the nursing staff, unless contraindicated by the physician.

Objectives:

- Maintain personal hygiene.

- Facilitate the transfer.

- Activate peripheral circulation and exercise the patient's muscles and limbs.

- Establish a good relationship with the patient.

- Observe the patient's general condition or pathological skin signs.

- Provide well-being and

comfort. Precautions:

- Measuring vital signs before bathing

- Protect the patient from accident and cold.

- Make sure that the water temperature is adequate.

- Avoid prolonged bathing

- Supply all necessary material

- Help the patient return to his unit

Material

- Bench or chair.

- Patient's wardrobe.

- Large and small towel.

- Personal hygiene items, lotion, deodorant, shampoo.

Procedure:

- Evaluate vital signs.

- Arrange the conditions for bathing.

- Orient the patient to urinate.

- Take the patient to the bathroom and adjust ventilation.

- Help the patient undress and maintain privacy.

- Facilitate everything for the patient to bathe himself, if he is able to do it, otherwise, it should be done by the nurse quickly to avoid body cooling.

- Start bathing with the face, then the head, thorax, upper extremities, back, abdomen, lower extremities, genitals and buttocks.

- provide the towel for drying or assist you, if necessary.

- Help the patient to get dressed and go back to the unit.

Bath in the riverbed. It consists of cleaning the skin with soap and water, in the patient who is partially or totally dependent.

Procedure. Place

the paraban.

Offer bedpan or bedpan, if the patient craves it.

- Wash hands and lower the Fowler (if not contraindicated).

- Remove the patient's clothing while maintaining patient privacy.

- Keep the patient covered with the sheet up to the shoulders.

- Place the clothes in the laundry cart, which should be at the foot of the bed.

- Set and check the water temperature.

Place one cloth in the container to be used to wash the patient and another cloth in the container to be used for rinsing.

- Place the rinse cloth in the form of a glove so that the extremities of the fingers are protected, in order to avoid injuring the skin with the fingernails.

- Soap the face, ears and neck, avoid soap penetrating into the eye if there is an eye condition, eye wash should be done before.

- Rinse and dry in the same way you lathered.

- Lower the sheet to the pubic region.

- Rinse the thorax insisting on infra mammary folds, the abdomen and both upper limbs (emphasizing on the armpits, elbow folds and interdigital spaces), rinse and dry in the same order.

- Cover the patient's chest.

- Place the patient in lateral decubitus to soap, rinse and dry the cervical region up to the buttocks.

- Turn the patient (dorsal decubitus) and keep the chest covered.

- Uncover the lower limbs and rinse both thighs and legs down to the ankles.
Wash and dry.

- Lather both feet, insist on the interdigital spaces, rinse and dry.

Technique for dressing and undressing

the patient Dressing - Covering the body

with clothing.

Costumes. Define the hors d'oeuvres that serve to cover the body from the hygienic point of view.

The clothing should be a poor conductor of heat so that the thermal changes with the outside environment are gradual to conserve and maintain body heat in winter and the warmer season to avoid the outside temperature.

Objective:

- Maintain personal hygiene, cover the body and promote patient comfort.

Precautions:

Avoid drafts

Precautions:

Have all the necessary material ready.

Be aware of the patient's state of consciousness. Use the size that best matches the patient's physical constitution.

- When it comes to dressing the patient, do it first by the wound or limited area.

Clothes should be wrinkle-free.

Applying body mechanics.

Material

Pajamas or night shirt.

Laundry basket or cart.

-Biombo (if

necessary).

Procedure:

- Place the paraban (if necessary).

- Place the patient in a seated or semi-sitting position, if the patient's condition permits.

- Uncover the sleeve of the pajamas or shirt, first removing one arm at a time.

-Same arm seen with pajamas or shirt.

- Proceed in the same way for the other upper limb.

Button the shirt.

-Remove the top sheet and open the pajama wedge.

-Orient the patient to bend the legs and elevate the buttocks, if the patient's situation allows it.

Lower the pants and remove them.

Place the pants neatly in the same way (first lower limb and then the other one).

4.5 Morning and evening care procedure

Morning care: care provided to partially or totally incapacitated patients in the early morning hours.

Objectives:

Clean, refresh and relax the patient.

Arrange the patient for small-lunch.

-Provide aesthetics.

Educate the patient on hygienic aspects.

To eliminate the accumulation of grease on the skin of the face, eye and nasal secretions.

Precautions:

Maintaining patient privacy.

Use water at a suitable temperature, according to the patient's habits.

Afternoon care: Care provided to the partially or totally incapacitated patient in the late afternoon.

Objective:

Meeting the patient's physical and psychological needs to promote restful sleep.

Precautions:

Maintaining patient privacy.

Do not massage the legs to avoid embolisms.

Observe the condition of the skin and sacral region before giving the massage (strengthening, cracks, other signs or damage).

Check dressings, ligatures and anti-embolism stockings, alter or adjust.

4.6 Feeding procedure for a palliative care patient

Nasogastric intubation: is the introduction of a tube through the nostrils or mouth into the stomach.

Objectives:

1. Establish the medical diagnosis.

2. Apply therapeutic measures.

3. Feeding the patient who cannot do it spontaneously.

4. Establish a means of draining gastric contents and extracting gases.

5. Prevent vomiting and abdominal distention

Precautions:

1) Have all the necessary material ready.

2) Be aware of the patient's state of consciousness.

3) Use the size that best matches the patient's physical constitution.

If possible, place the patient in a seated or semi-sitting position; if the patient is unconscious in Trendelenburg position, leaning on the left side in ventral decubitus. This position prevents bronchial aspiration.

4) Moisten the probe with distilled water or saline solution, avoiding dripping, never with greasy substances, to avoid irritation of the mucous membranes and bronchial aspiration.

5) Ask the patient which nostril he/she breathes best, and pass the probe through the nostril with the greatest difficulty.

6) If the individual presents any nasal alteration, such as a deviated septum, which prevents passing the probe through the nasal cavity, introduce it through the mouth after removing the dental prosthesis.

7) If the person is unconscious, tilt the chin to the chest to close the trachea and push the probe between breaths to make sure it did not stop the trachea.

8)Watch for signs of tracheal entry, choking or labored breathing in a conscious person and cyanosis in an unconscious person or without cough reflex. If these signs are present, immediately remove the tube, allow the patient to rest and try again.

9) To check the correct placement of the tube, never insert the end of the tube into the water. If the tube is in the trachea, the patient may inhale water; and in any case, the absence of bubbling does not confirm correct placement, as the tube may be swollen in the trachea or esophagus.

10) Check that the tube is in the stomach.

11) Measuring gastric contents

Material:

1) Tray or side table.

2) Gastric tube (Latex, silicone, with

balloon 3) Towel, cloth, or slip.

Feeding probe

Feeding tube: The introduction of liquid or melted food through a tube that passes through the nose or mouth to the stomach.

Objective:

Maintain adequate patient nutritional status

Precautions:

Ensure the hygienic condition of the oral and nasal cavities.

Aspirate before food administration and observe the characteristics of the extracted substances.

If the aspirated content is greater than 100 ml, do not feed the patient and inform the physician.

Measure the amount of food and water administered, providing them at an adequate temperature.

Gravity feed management

Alter the probe with current standards of hygiene and epidemiology, to avoid damaging the hydrochloric acid in the stomach and causing an unnecessary response.

Avoid sudden movements that may cause vomiting to the patient, once given food.

Material

Gastric tube (Levine, among

others). Towel, cloth or shelter.

Containers for

garbage. Glass with

water.

Adhesive, blade to fix the

probe. Scissors.

Spatulas.

Buy.

Paper towels or napkin. Stethoscope.

20 ml syringe, feeding syringe, funnel or disposable feeding bag.

Mounted clamp.

Container with food

Container with water

Bladder catheterization procedure for patients with difficulty in urinary elimination that would require palliative care.

Bladder catheterization is the introduction of a catheter or catheter through the meatus and urethral canal to the inside of the bladder.

Objectives:

Bladder emptying.

Determine if urine deficit is caused by retention urinary obstruction, or anuria.

To obtain urine samples for the study.

Emptying the bladder prior to major surgery to avoid surgical trauma to the organ level and the patient urinating in the operating room to cause sphincter relaxation.

Precautions:

Make cleaning of the genital organs to reduce bacteria at that level and avoid being dragged in from the bladder.

Do not force the catheter to pass, to avoid trauma to the urethra, keep in mind the caliber of the catheters for the type of urethra;

Ask the patient to cough during insertion, as this will facilitate the insertion of the probe.

After finishing the procedure, the uncircumcised male should be careful to push the foreskin over the glans.

In the case of the Foley probe, fix it with saline solution (no air, no glucose solutions).

If the catheter remains fixed, clamp it periodically to regain bladder tone.

If urine is retained, allow outflow up to 400 ml every 30 minutes, allow outflow of 200 ml to avoid rapid stagnation of urine.

Change of probes according to service

standards. Equipment

Compresses.

Waste container.

Sterile syringe with saline solution.

Band-aid (stays on permanently).

Scissors (remains permanent).

Saco collector (remains

permanent). Paraban (if

necessary).

Bowel elimination procedure in a palliative care patient
Emollient Enemas. When there is severe constipation, painful anal disorder or

irritation of the intestinal mucosa, a fatty enema may be appropriate. The oil acts mainly as a lubricant to facilitate evacuation. Various oils can be used, such as mineral, oil, cottonseed and others. The amount used is small, usually 150 to 200 ml and usually the patient is asked to hold the enema for about 1 hr. Many times, after a retention enema, a cleansing enema is indicated.

Precautions:

o Administer cleansing enema beforehand, to keep the colon free of feces.
o Hold it 10-20 M.
o Apply lubricant to the anal and perianal region and to the inner thighs if an anthelmintic enema is to be performed.
o Retention enemas should be scheduled before meals, because a full stomach can stimulate peristalsis.
o Retention enema with oil should not be administered before cleansing enema, but do it 1 hour after the fatty enema, recommended to be soap and water to help expel the stool completely softened.
o In anti-parasitic enemas, once administered, should be followed by cleansing enema.
o If the sphincter is not functional, place a balloon rectal catheter.
o Complications may occur from the enema being retained.

Material:

o General Enema Equipment.
o He added the indicated medication, gloves and a syringe to measure the medication, if necessary.

Procedure for administering oxygen to palliative care patients. Oxygen by nasal whisker

Metal support. Metal fixation with a fork with two recess hooks (allowing the oxygen bill), slightly concave to be placed on the nostrils.

Plastic fork. Hollow plastic attachment with two short, straight extensions, perfectly attachable to the nose.

Objective: To apply whisker oxygen therapy when the patient has difficulty accepting the catheter.

Precautions:

- Observe the technical condition of the mustache (that it is not obstructed).
- Fix the mustache on the head, by edge or gauze, never for behind, which causes discouragement for the patient lying down.

CHAPTER 5:
COMMUNICATION

Communication is the transmission of information from one subject to another, it is the act of communicating as a process through which ideas are transmitted in order to inform and modify behavior. There are elements that influence this process such as noise, context, filters. In healthcare, professional work includes the establishment of direct interpersonal relationships, which go beyond the simple interaction between two individuals. The therapeutic relationship that is created between nurse and patient is achieved by establishing common goals, collaborative relationships and exchange of mutual help, from a holistic perception. From the beginnings of nursing, Florence Nightingale already pronounced the importance and necessity of communication in nurse-patient relationships, years later H. Pepla u considered communication as the nursing method. And in the same way both Dorothea Orem and Virginia Henderson developed their theory in some way with the psychosocial sphere and proposed the development of personal relationships involving communicative influence. The objective of communication is the transmission of a message between sender and receiver and that both share a meaning. Health personnel must know how to listen in order to be able to understand the patient, so that optimal communication improves the quality of life and satisfaction of both patients and their families.

Language characterizes the human being, so it is impossible not to communicate. There are different elements that make up the communicative act such as:

- Message: The message that the sender intends to convey to the receiver.
- Sender: The person who chooses the message to be communicated.
- Receiver: It is the one who decodes the message and offers a response.
- Channel: The means by which the message is received, where great importance is given to the sense organs.
- Transmitter: It is the form in which the message is transmitted, it can be written,

oral, visual, auditory.

There are many ways to establish communication, the verbal is the most frequent is in which the person consciously chooses the words that depends on the cultural and social characteristics, but it is also important what is transmitted, not only with words but with gestures, expressions and is where the observation acquires a prominent role, 80% of communication involves body movements, gestures and physical appearance. In our profession it is not only about observing signs and symptoms but also about recognizing the response to our actions. The current culture of care and the integration of user satisfaction into the health care system has an impact on our responsibility as professionals to improve quality. This implies a real change in the meaning of care and quality of care.

5.1 Factors that distort communication

The interruption of the communicative process brings with it the achievement or non-achievement of the proposed objectives.

- Ability to communicate. The nursing staff must have a clear, simple language, low and soft tone.
- Perceptions: Respect both personal perceptions and those of the individual family and the community.
- Personal space: Perform each task at the appropriate place and time improvisations that may affect the communicative process.
- Territoriality: The nursing professional has to be located in time, space and be tactful at the moment of carrying out the communicative process since the territoriality where the process is executed can intervene positively and negatively.
- Functions and relationships: If the functions attributed to each person are not fully complied with and if the relationships are fractured for any reason from the first impact, it may cause irreversible damage to the communicative process.
- Time: It must be planned, not to be exceeded so that the communicative process

becomes an exhausting space.

- The environment: Maintaining a balanced environment helps the understanding and development of the communicative process.

- Emotions and self-esteem. The psychological aspect influences both positively and negatively the communicative process, so the nursing staff must incorporate the knowledge acquired in medical psychology to avoid damage and harm to patients and that contribute to frustrate the communicative process and thus the rupture, loss or deviation of the proposed objectives.

Influence of nurse-patient communication on rehabilitation.

Communication, when the objectives established for it are met, is an important element in therapeutic support, so that the nursing staff requires training in communication skills so that their practical activity is closely related to emotional accompaniment and coping possibilities, It is important to point out the attitudes of trust as a key aspect in the nurse-patient relationship, the harmonious climate of solidarity, the use of accessible language, taking into account the information needs of the families, dedicating sufficient time and using a protocol of care agreed upon by the professional team makes communication effective and therefore provides a tool for the improvement in the quality of care.

Communication with the family

The nursing staff in their communication with the family focuses on providing the families with the necessary social skills to establish adequate and effective communication; they should be trained in patient care. When notified of bad news, the family usually reacts with stupor and denial, there is a great family impact and the disease becomes the focus of the activity of all the members. Open communication between the health care team and the family facilitates the process by which they adapt to the different family events and are given the opportunity for family participation in the patient's care.

The nursing professional's communication with the family must comply with the following aspects:

➤ Provide clear information to families about the disease and where to go.

➤ To ensure that the patient is receiving the care he/she needs at each stage.

➤ Involve them in patient care.

➤ Offer emotional and physical psychological support.

➤ To accompany in the stage of agony and bereavement.

➤ The professional must adopt a helpful posture at all times.

➤ Care must be taken with verbal and non-verbal language

➤ Avoid showing haste in conversations.

➤ The verbal message must be clear and avoid ambiguity.

Nursing professional communication with the patient.

➤ Communicate to the patient who you are, what you do and who the members of the health care team are.

➤ Recognize the patient by name and know what they prefer to be called.

➤ Be close to the patient, give confidence.

➤ Make eye contact.

5.2 Health communication techniques

Technical communication is the process of transmitting technical information through writing, speech and other means of communication to a specific audience.

• Lecture: Consists of a brief conference where specific topics are presented. Advantages of the talk.

• It is economical because for its execution it is enough with the one that exposes it.

• It requires little time.

• You read to many people at the same time.

• Subsequent meetings can be derived from it.

Disadvantages

• It is not suitable for changing negative habits and attitudes, since the subjects who listen remain passive, purely receptive.

The talk should not be abused because it may appear tired and the population may lose interest, its use is advisable in health promotion and prevention, it plays an important role in health emergencies, it is useful for a rumor that is limiting adequate attitudes towards population health.

Demonstration

It is a technique where action and words are combined. The person who performs the action at the same time explains. It is efficient because it is an audiovisual way, a dynamic vision is obtained and it creates motivation.

The panel

A group of people present a topic in front of an audience that then participates with questions and answers.

This technique is most appropriate for prevention, recovery and health rehabilitation.

Round Table

It differs from the panel in that the level reached by the science on the subject to be discussed does not allow for agreement.

This technique is recommended to be used preferably in prevention, recovery and rehabilitation.

The interview.

Planned conversation can be individual or group It

has 3 main objectives

• Collecting information
• Providing information
• Modify negative attitudes that predict health. Group
dynamics

It is a dynamic process where topics and tasks are analyzed collectively and opinions and suggestions are discussed, this discussion makes each member aware of their own limitations, stereotypes and prejudices.

CHAPTER 6:

COMMUNITY HEALTH PROMOTION AND PREVENTION

The phenomenon of providing care is as old as the beginning of life. Care is innate in human beings; man, like all living beings, has always had the need to care, to maintain the continuity of life and, of course, to do so in a way that is conscientious and oriented towards human well-being.

Uniting knowledge and care, but we cannot do without either. Governments spend most of the health budget on curing and rehabilitating   people, ignoring   the value   of health education, which sets the tone in maintaining health and in the knowledge of healthy actions to maintain it. Therefore, in the training of health professionals, they should be instructed in the transmission of knowledge in the communities and during their training process, they should be offered the necessary tools to be able to improve the quality of life of the inhabitants of the communities and work on the basis of prevention in health issues. That is why the preparation of the citizens is necessary. A country in which the citizens perform tasks with quality of e x c e l e n c e , is a prepared nation. A society is prepared when all or most of its citizens are prepared; an individual is prepared when he is able to face the problems that arise in his job and solve them. Thus, the concept of preparedness expresses the problem, the starting point of pedagogical science and its category.

Nursing is considered the art of caring, a profession endowed with a body of knowledge   that makes this care offered by the professionals of this career to be intelligent care. Therefore, one must learn how to educate so that this care meets the expected objective. For this, the nursing professional must have an integral multidisciplinary formation, be trained with pedagogical and   didactic bases , notions of philosophy, sociology, psychology, anthropology, ethics, bioethics, basic sciences of foundation and the own contents of the nursing discipline if they will be able to develop the educational competence with an integral approach, solving situations and problems that will make the effectiveness of the action. This requires a reflective-comprehensive effort and the elaboration of applied theoretical and applied models that enable a better interpretation of the task. The education in the process of formation of the person must be adapted to these essential characteristics. Every person has the right to reach his or her maximum development or self-realization. The p s i c o l o g i c a l perspective analyzes the differences between individuals, both qualitative and quantitative, in the various dimensions of the person: heredity, specific capacities, attitudes, interests and values, individual and social behavior. This principle is called individualized teaching and is the set of methods and techniques that allow acting simultaneously on several people, adapting the work to the development of their aptitudes and development.

Florence N i g h t i n g i n g a l e initiated nursing research and was the first to write about the discipline. Since that time, nursing has been about providing care and educating the individual to maintain his or her health in the best possible condition.

6.1 Nursing fields of action in health education

The fields of action of nursing affect all health processes, providing education for health in each of them, and this is a situation to be addressed in the professional training process of the nurse.

Health education is one of the activities performed by the nursing professional, an activity learned during the career. And that becomes indispensable in the act of taking care of people's health and life. With the beginning of the world or Christianity has given rise to a humanitarian approach to the churches. In the c o n t r a
The reform, continues this referent, to the orders of religious leaders such as the Daughters of Charity, whose work in caring for the sick left two principles that have become primary care nurses day and night:

In general, historically, the nursing activity arises as something primitive but inherent to the human quality of the women who practiced it and in doing so, began to exercise a relationship of interdependence with the person subject of care, where, as can be seen, the transfer of knowledge for the preservation of health began,   thus initiating the educational processes of care for the person receiving care. Subsequently, th e basis of professional nursing was established when Florence Nightingale, in her Notes on Nursing (1998) tried define the specific contribution of nursing to health care. In the theoretical development of nursing, concepts and propositions are considered that propose the relationships between **them**, which have been called meta paradigms. The meta paradigmatic concepts that make up the conceptual framework of nursing and that are present in all nursing models, such as the models of Orem, Henderson, Roy, Rogers, Johnson, King and Levine, are: The person, health, environment, and nursing care.

CHAPTER 7:

SYNTHESIS OF NURSING THEORIES AND MODELS APPLIED TO COMMUNITY CARE

Nursing is also a professionwith a university degree that is dedicated to the integral care of the individual, the family and the community in all stages of the life cycle and in their development processes. In Spain and Colombia there is another ofice within Nursing whose functions complement the work of nurses: the titled technician in auxiliary nursing care, better known as nursing assistant.

Nursing modelsand theories are intended to describe, establish and examine the phenomena that shape the practice of GeneralNursing.

It is assumed by the discipline that in order to determine that a nursing theory exists, it must contain the elements of the Meta paradigm of nursing.

Each discipline makes terms related to theory and its development its own in order to provide it with a body of knowledge to guide the practice of the discipline.

7.1 Types of models

Each author groups the models according to his or her own criteria. They are usually based on the role that nursing plays in providing care. Thus, we can divide them into:

• Naturalistic models.

• Substitution or assistance models.

•Interrelationship

  models. Naturalistic

  models

Its main representative is Florence Nightingale. In 1859 she tries to define the nature of nursing care in her book Notes on nursing; "There is a tendency to believe that medicine cures. Nothing is less true, medicine is the surgery of functions as true surgery is the surgery of organs, neither one nor the other cures, only nature can cure.

41

- What nursing care does in both cases is to restore the patient to full health.

7.2 Florence Nightingale's theory

He had understood the need to have a reference scheme, a conceptual framework. From this first attempt at conceptualization, until this question was formally asked again, almost a century passed. It is the simplest of all the models, where he stated that nursing knowledge differed greatly from the knowledge of medical sciences and made clear the role of the nurse.

He pointed out that one of the results of nursing is to preserve the vital energy of the patient, he stated that cleanliness, ventilation and food were essential elements for the recovery of the patient and defined a concept of health in a state of well-being that translates into taking advantage of the energies of people. He differentiates between healthy and sick people when he proposes measures to control the environment to preserve health.

Substitution or assistance models

The role of nursing consists of replacing or helping to carry out the actions that the person is unable to perform at some point in his or her life, actions that preserve life, both by encouraging self-careon the part of the person.

The two most important representatives of this trend are Virginia Hendersonand Dorothea Orem.

Interrelationship models

In these models, the nurse's role is to promote the adaptation of the person in a changing environment, fostering either the interpersonal relationship (nurse-patient) or the patient's relationship with his or her environment.

The most representative models are those of HildegardePeplau, CallistaRoy, MarthaE. Rogers and Myra Levine. Rogersand Myra Levine.

7.3 Virginia Henderson Model

Theoretical basis

- It is a modelofsubstitutionorassistance.

- Part of Maslow's concept of human needs.

The human being is a biopsychosocialbeingwith needs that he/she tries to meet independently according to his/her habits, culture, etc. The human being has 14 basic needs:

Breathing, eating and drinking, evacuating, moving and maintaining posture, sleeping and resting, dressing and undressing, maintaining body temperature, keeping clean, avoiding hazards, communicating, worshipping, working, playing and learning.

Healthis a person's ability to carry out all those activities that allow him/her to maintain his/her basic needs satisfied.

The human being should also be viewed from a

biopsychosocial, spiritual and holistic perspective, different in their feelings and emotions. The overload of work in hospital units makes this care increasingly difficult. Let us remember that those of us who offer our nursing services do not make value judgments, we empathize and accompany until the last breath.

Methodology of care

It consists of a care plan: a problem-solving process. The human being should be seen from a biopsychosocial, spiritual and holistic perspective, with different feelings and emotions. The overload of work in hospital units makes it increasingly difficult to provide this care as such. let us remember that those of us who offer our nursing services do not make value judgments, and accompany until the last breath.

7.4 Model of Dorothea Orem

Theoretical basis

- It is a model of substitution or assistance.

  - Maslow's theory of human needs.

  - General systems theory.

Assumptions and values

For Dorothea Orem, the human being is an organism that is biological, psychological, and in interaction with its environment, to which it is subject. It has the capacity to create, communicate, and perform beneficial activities for itself and for others.

Health is a state that signifies structural and functional integrity that is achieved through universal actions called self-care I conceptualize the proper role of the nurse in attending to the healthy and sick person in their activities to contribute to their health or recovery .I state that nursing performance depends on the physician and that human beings have basic needs that must be met and are normally covered by the healthy individual.

Self-care is a human need that constitutes every action that human beings perform through their values, beliefs, etc. in order to maintain life, health and well-being. They are deliberate actions that require learning. When the person is unable to carry out these actions on his or her own, either due to limitation or disability, a situation of self-care dependence arises.

There are three types of self-care:

Those derived from the fundamental needs of each individual: eating, drinking, breathing, ...

Those derived from the specific needs that arise at certain
moments of development: childhood, adolescence, adulthood

and old age.

7.5 Peplau Model

Model established by the nurse HildegardPeplau

Theoretical basis

- Interrelationship model.

- Psychoanalytic theory.

- Theory of human needs

- Concept of motivation.

- Concept of personal development.

- Orientation phase. The patient attempts to clarificate his or her dificulties and the extent of the need for help. The nurse assesses the person's situation

- Identification phase. The patient clarifies his or her situation, identifies the need for help and responds to the people who offer help. The nurse makes the diagnosisof the situation and formulates the careplan.

- Utilization phase. The patient makes use of the nursing services and gets the maximum benefit from them. The nurse implements the careplan, thus helping the person and herself to grow to maturity.

- Resolution phase. The patient resumes independence. The nurse assessesthe growth that has occurred between the two.

Nursing functions: In Hildegarde Peplau's model, they consist of helping the human being to mature personally by facilitating a creative, constructive and productive life.

7.6 Callista Roy Model

Methodology of care

Nursing care process.Callista Roy's model Adaptation theory.

Assumptions and values: The human being is a biopsychosocial being - in constant interaction with the environment. This inter-action is carried out through adaptation which, for Roy, consists in the adaptation of the 4 spheres of life:

- Physiological area. Circulation, temperature, oxygen, fluids, sleep, activity, nutrition and elimination.

- Self-image area. The image one has of oneself.

- Role domain area. The different roles that a human being fulfills throughout his or her life.

- Area of independence. Positive interactions with his environment, in this case, the people with whom he exchanges influences that procure a balance of his self-image and role mastery.

The human being, in turn, is at a certain point in what he calls the "health-illness continuum. This point may be closer to health or disease by virtue of the capacity of each individual to respond to the stimuli he receives from his environment. If he responds positively, adapting, he will approach a state of health, otherwise he will become ill.

Health is a state and a process of being and becomes integrated and global. This can be modified by environmental stimuli, which for Callista are.

- Focal stimuli. Precipitating changes that have to be dealt with. For example, a flu process.

- Contextual stimuli. All those that are present in the process. For example, ambient temperature.

- Residual stimuli. These are values and beliefs from past experiences, which may have influence on the present situation. For example, shelter, home treatments.

7.7 Martha Rogers Model

Theoretical basis

- Interrelationship model.

- General systems theory

- Evolutionary theory.

Assumptions and values: The human being is a unified whole in constant relationship with its environment, with which it exchanges matter and energy; and which differs from other living beings by its capacity to change this environment and to make choices that allow it to develop as a person. For Rogers, the human being is an energy field in interaction with another energy field: the environment. This is evidenced by the principles of thermodynamics, on which his theoretical framework is based. The constant flux of waves between people and the environment are the basis of nursing activities. Life is a flux of experiences. To be alive is to become irreversibly more complex, diverse and differentiated-nothing is ever again what it has been. The capacity to do, describes the way in which beings interact with their environment to actualize their potentials that allow them to develop and participate, therefore, in the creation of human and environmental reality. Health is the constant harmonic maintenance of human beings with their environment. If harmony is broken, health and well-being disappear.

Nursing functions In this model, the aim is for the individual to reach his or her maximum health potential.

CHAPTER 8:
ACCIDENTS IN THE HOME

The word Accident has Latin origin, accident, which means chance. The WHO considers that an accident is a fortuitous event, generally unfortunate or harmful, independent of human will, caused by an external force acting rapidly and manifested by the appearance of organic lesions or mental disorders. They are the fifth leading cause of death in the world.

Domestic accidents are those that occur in the dwelling itself, patios, gardens, garages, access to apartments, stairway lobbies. All places belonging to the home. It is in the home, where the family usually spends most of its time throughout its life, and it is there where there are possibilities of any kind of domestic accident. Although all members of the family are equally likely to suffer an accident, it is children and the elderly who suffer most frequently. Their age and their situation in life make them, due to their ignorance, carelessness, weakness and mental characteristics, the most defenseless and vulnerable.

8.1 Most common accidents

The number of accident victims is increasing every year, and these accidents are the leading causes of death worldwide, many of which are avoidable and preventable. In the reviews carried out, the main causes of accidents at different ages are:

- Falls
- Wounds
- Burns
- Ingestion of toxic substances
- Choking
- Electrocution

8.2 General causes

A causal analysis of the occurrence of accidents reveals general elements that make the occurrence of accidents possible, such as:

- Low illumination
- Wet, damp, slippery floors
- Very high or narrow steps
- Running down the stairs
- Climbing on chairs or other objects
- High beds
- Poisoning with liquids and powders
- Electrical cables
- Carpets
- Inadequate handling of household appliances
- Fire by candles
- Gas emergency.
- Concave bathtubs
- Containers with water in which a small child can be submerged.
- Plants with small fruits that can be ingested or introduced in orifices.
- Poorly plugged wells
  Most frequent causes in children
- Cradle
- Bed
- Bathroom
- Dining room
- Street
- Field
  Most frequent causes in older adults
- Falls

- Wounds

- Fractures

The risk of the older adult is over-added since the use of psychotropic drugs or other CNS depressants and osteomyoarticular conditions, visual deficit and balance disorders led to the precipitation of accidents, as well as structural problems in the home and the presence of objects on the floor. Most of the older adults have little knowledge about the causes of accidents, much less the behavior to follow in the event of an accident.

It is important to mention the dangers of technology, which can cause physical and emotional damage in some stages of life, submerging them in illnesses such as depression, anxiety and low self-esteem because it does not allow them to develop the necessary skills to demonstrate the qualities and tools that each one has.

We also have biological hazards of food origin such as bacteria, viruses and parasites. These organisms are frequently associated with handlers and contaminated raw products that are accidentally introduced into humans.

8.3 Activities to prevent accidents at home

The nurse in his community intervention, being aware of the main causes of the occurrence of accidents, will make an action plan involving activities easily understood by the inhabitants of the community in his charge and that will help to raise the perception of risk in the homes and surroundings and contribute to the reduction of accidents. We can mention some of them.

1. Keep small objects and toys out of reach of children that can be put in the mouth or nose and cause choking.
2. Cut food into small pieces and be supervised by adults.
3. Do not neglect the baby while breastfeeding
4. Avoid child's play with plastic bags.

Inside the house

1 Rehearse an evacuation plan in case of fire.

2 Placing locks on cabinets, to prevent children from accessing harmful
   substances

3 Keep electrical cables out of the reach of children.

4 Place plates over electrical outlets to avoid electrocution.

5 Keep hazardous chemicals out of reach of children and heat sources.

6 Do not use soft drink containers to store toxic substances.

7 Prepare medicine cabinet out of children's reach

8 Fit accessories on doors to prevent them from closing suddenly.

9 Not having stairs without handrails.

10 Use rugs in bathrooms to prevent slipping

11If you are an older adult, keep a lamp near the bed to turn on when you get up.

12The use of the cane in the elderly.

13Keep objects such as knives, needles, scissors, etc., in safe places.

14If physical exertion is required, it should be performed with knees bent, back
   straight and feet slightly apart to avoid muscle tears or contractures.

15Avoid having the children's play area in the kitchen

16Keep the iron out of reach of children

17 Place safety gates at the top and bottom of the stairs

18Identify the risk points in your home that could cause an accident in order to
   reduce them.

8.4 The role of the community health professional in the prevention of accidents.

Nursing as a profession encompasses the care of a society and its relationship with its environment where the surrounding conditions are taken into account for the formulation of strategies according to the identified needs.

The clinical, community and administrative environment has become a virtuous circle where nurses have exercised their knowledge, highlighting personal care as a differential factor in the execution of daily activities.

Strengthening community nursing practices in order to reduce the occurrence of accidents are social objectives and the challenges that are posed in community nursing is fundamental for nursing care. The community nurse should promote programs for the prevention of accidents in the home allowing with his work to increase the levels of knowledge of caregivers and promote actions aimed at obtaining a safer environment, assess the impact and reduction of potential dangers of accidents in families and thus raise the quality of life of the people in their care in the community. Taking into account that the main medicine is prevention, health promotion actions should be strengthened in primary health care, the community nurse should carry out a multidisciplinary and intersectorial work in order to guarantee a healthy environment without risks of accidents and with them achieve a healthy community. The responsibilities of the nursing professional are immersed in the pedagogical assistance administrative activities where several tools are implemented to help provide the proposed action in each case.

From a broad perspective, the nursing profession applied in a community environment is supported by the WHO through the strategy created for the preservation of healthy environments where the theoretical, axiological and moral bases of the profession are founded, making it a fundamental link of the global chain of interactions to communities that strengthens the functioning of health systems. The nursing professional in the field of health and safety applies knowledge and tools within the community in order to promote, maintain and improve the health of the population. Leadership in this discipline allows directing and coordinating the different processes or health plans in any environment such as community.

Nursing staff tools

> Instrumental: The use of the Nursing Care Process, a perfect tool for planning care that impacts the health of the individual, the family and the community.
> Personal: In the management implemented by the nursing professional: active listening is a tool to attend and understand the subject of care, establishing a relationship of trust that leads to the creation of habits of care and risk prevention.
> Systematic: The innate leadership of the nurse provides characteristics of adaptation to different environments to achieve the design of programs for the improvement of the community environment, fostering family bonding and guiding families in the adoption of good practices.
> Specific: Relating the theories and skills of the nurse, structured care plans are generated through a methodology under the concepts of the profession, which are unique and indispensable to achieve the proposed objectives.

These nursing tools allow to achieve the goals of care where some nursing theorists such as Orem, Watson, and Lenninger are used in the management process and that through the implementation of the Meta paradigm: person, environment, health and nursing, are involved in the process of nursing care to meet the care needs of individuals, families and communities.

Nurses must empower and visualize their managerial role within the communities. This will enable it to have greater relevance within the different social groups. and also facilitates better management of tasks, crises and situations that arise in the community.

The nexus of nursing leadership should be networked so as to demonstrate that professionals are in constant interaction. Community work is focused on health promotion, achieving teamwork, innate roles, interpersonal relationships, the subject of care with the interaction in the community and families, achieving the generation of knowledge through health education and risk prevention, which are impacted by the tools already mentioned.

BIBLIOGRAPHY

1. Attention to the Elderly. Grupo de trabajo del anciano de la semFYC, Ediciones Eurobook, SL. Madrid 1997:11-47.

2. C. De Alba Romero, J. M. Baena Díez, M. C. de Hoyos Alonso, A. Gorroñogoitia Iturbe, C. Litargo Gil, L. Martín.

3. Muñoz, A ECS From health promotion to healthy work environments, Workers' Health 18(2) 141-152 [Online]; 2010 [cited 2019, Available from: http://wwwscieloorgve/scielophp?script=sci_ar

4. Torres C, Perception of nursing care quality in hospitalized oncology patients Cuidarte magazine 2(2) 138-148 [Online]; 2011 Available from: https://wwwrevistacuidarteorg/indexphp/cuidarte/article/view/49/688.

5. Delgado A, The act of nursing care as a foundation for professional and research work Avances En Enfermería 33(3) 412-419 [Online]; 2015, Available from:https://searchproquestcom/docview/1819126028?accountid=47900

6. Muñoz, A ECS From health promotion to healthy work environments, Workers' Health 18(2) 141-152 [Online]; 2010 [cited 2019, Available from: http://wwwscieloorgve/scielophp?script=sci_ar

7. Torres C, Perception of nursing care quality in hospitalized oncology patients Cuidarte magazine 2(2) 138-148 [Online]; 2011 Available from: https://wwwrevistacuidarteorg/indexphp/cuidarte/article/view/49/688

8. Vega F Ramirez, The role of communication campaigns in health promotion and injury prevention in occupational health1(2)137-154 Retrieved July 12, 2018[Online];2010Available from: http://wwwaecses/1_2_comunicacion%20salud%20laboralpdf.

9. SegüelPalmaF   ,ELTrabajodelprofesionaldeenfermería : revisión de la literatura Ciencia y enfermería 21(2) 11-20 [Online]; 2015, Available from: https://scieloconicytcl/scielophp?pid=S0717-95532015000200002&script=sci_arttext.

10. Tokur M, Using the Omaha System in Occupational Health Nursing

Applications: Advantages of a Common Language in the Diagnosis Intervention and Evaluation of Nurses Health Problems Revista Elsevier Volume 152 (7) 488-494[Online]; 2014 Available from: https://wwwsciencedirectcom/science/article/pii/S1877042814053051

11. Albornoz Mancera, D.M. (2009). The importance of transcultural dad in nursing knowledge. Rev Paraninfo Digital, 3 (7), Available at: </para/n7/100d. php>. Accessed January 24, 2014.

12. Artigas Lelong, B., Vennasar Veny, M. (2009). Health in the 21st century: the challenge of multicultural care.

13. González Juárez, L., Noreña Peña, A.L. (2011). Intercultural communication as a means to favor culturally acceptable care. Rev ENEO-UNAM, 8(1), 55-60.

14. Benavides M. Preventable accidents: Children's injuries and their relationships with social and family environments. Espacio Para La Infancia 2012; 18:29-31.

15. Bustos E, Cabrales G, Cerón M, Naranjo Y. Epidemiology of accidental injuries in children: Review of international and national statistics. Bol Med Hosp Infant Mex 2014; 71(2):68-75.

16. Gorrita RR, Barrientos G, Gorrita Y. Risk factors, family functioning and unintentional injuries in children under five years of age. Havana Journal of Medical Sciences 2016; 22(1):42-57.

17. Martínez M, Gutiérrez H, Alonso M, Hernández L. Knowledge of a group of mothers on the prevention of accidents at home. Re- view of Medical Sciences of Havana 2015; 21(2):335-345.

18. Cedrés A, Morosini F, Margni C, López A, Alegretti M, Dall'Orso P, et al. Animal bites in children. What is the current situation in the Pediatric?

19. Emergency Department at Pereira Rossell Hospital? Arch Pediatr Urug 2018; 89(1):15-20. DOI: http://dx.doi.org/10.31134/ap.89.1.3.

20. Garzón N. Unintentional injuries a public health problem. Bogotá D.C: National Institute of Legal Medicine; 2015.

21. Torres M, Fonseca C, Díaz Martínez M, del Campo O, Roché R. Accidents in

childhood: A current problem in pediatrics. MEDISAN 2010.

22. Cardero E, Mojena G, Porto Y, del Río L, Calas G. Clinicotherapeutic characterization of children and adolescents with Aero digestive foreign bodies. MEDISAN 2018; 22(4):384-393.

23. Olmedo M.C.; Systematics for the protocolization of nursing care. Revista de Calidad Asistencial (online). 2010. (May 02, 2012); No.25.

24. Colliére MF. Promoting life. Mexico: Mc Graw-Hill In- teramericana; 1993.

25. Ministry of Health. Interinstitutional Nursing Commission. Evaluation of the quality of nursing services, 2002.

26. Peña K, Rodríguez J. Nursing in the face of the chaos and complexity approach. Cultura de cuidados. 2003; 14:79-82.

27. Collective of authors, Family and Social Nursing, Chapters 18. Editorial Ciencias Médicas de la Habana, Cuba 2004.

28. Álvarez Sintes, Temas de Medicina General Integral, Volume II, chapter 15. Editorial Ciencias Médicas de la Habana, Cuba 2001.

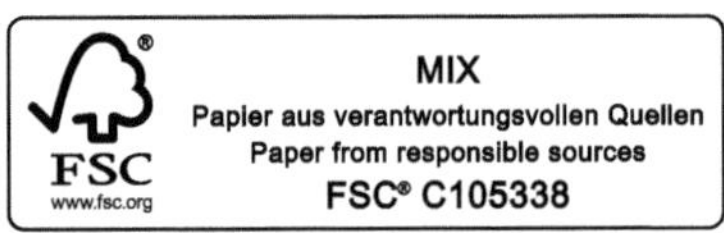

Printed by Books on Demand GmbH, Norderstedt / Germany